*"Why is it that our memory is good
enough to retain the least triviality that happens to us,
and yet not good enough to recollect how often
we have told it to the same person?"*

-François de La Rochefoucauld (1613-1680)

# ISBN-13: 978-1518737763
# ISBN-10: 1518737765

**Order at Amazon to get additional copies of**

The Alzheimer's Memory Hole has a Silver Lining*

Rome and the Vatican Easy Sightseeing*

Florence Easy Sightseeing

Venice Easy Sightseeing

A Woodpecker in his Leg*

Voice Power*

After Your First Six Words, I Know You


* Available in Kindle

# The ALZHEIMER'S
## MEMORY HOLE
## HAS A SILVER LINING

You Can Prevent, Minimize or Survive
Alzheimer's

By Donald H. Bowling, M.Ed.

*"You've got to accentuate the positive*
*Eliminate the negative*
*And latch on to the affirmative*
*don't mess with Mister In-Between."*
    -Johnny Mercer

# Summary Of Contents

From the Author; Don Bowling

My experiences, both remembered by me and a memory hole recorded by my daughter.

## Chapter 1: A Gigantic Snake
- Hallucinations are real to the person who sees or hears them.
- Alzheimer memory holes exclude all memories without any residues.

- Pet scans exhibit the brain damage by amyloid plaques and tau protein tangles, the causes of Alzheimer's.
- Regular "old-age problems," also occur and sometimes Parkinson's disease.
- Meditation offers the ability to manage stress, that is one of the causes of Alzheimer's.

- I move to Aegis senior facility. I live in their memory treatment unit.
- The program is centered on the "Best Friends" approach.
- Memory habilitation, communication and brain exercises are conducted.

- They are all like snowflakes, each one is different.
- Grouping for treatment is difficult.

- Namenda is one effective treatment for my memory and stopping dementia.
- Author volunteers for treating fellow residents so I may understand Alzheimer's.
- Treatment programs described by me, the retired teacher.
- Daughter informs me that she kept a journal of my behavior and treatment during my five months of a memory hole.

# From the Author

I am a retired school principal and teacher of the handicapped. Last year, I saw a gigantic snake and was attacked by a disease called Alzheimer's. It wasn't so simple because the snake was a hallucination from Lewy-Body dementia connected to Parkinson's disease. If you want to see what my life was like before the gigantic snake, turn to the appendix.

For now I want to tell you about how I survived this five-month hole in my memory and hope that you, a relative or friends will see how my memory hole had a silver lining.

This book is mainly written in present tense because it helped me when my helpers focused on the present moment. As a dementia patient it freed me to deal with the successes and defeats of the present. Not to grieve about the problems of the past and fears toward the future. That may only work for me, but my biggest obstacles were the memory holes with which I had to deal.

I wish to thank God and the many people who helped me emerge with a new personality gained from my bout with the disease and old age. I thank my daughter and son who supported me during 2014 and 2015, Tania and Rosita who prepared me each day for life in Aegis' assisted living and memory care facility, the total staff of Aegis Napa who allowed me to make my home in their wonderful environment, the makers of Namenda, a drug that reduced the Amyloid Plaques or Tau Tangles in my brain, and the medical people including Dr. Gary Small MD of UCLA, my alma mater, who through his book, *The Alzheimer's Prevention Program*, brought me to a new life.

My role as a resident of an eldercare facility does not give me access to the medical records of residents of whom I write my experiences and I always consider their privacy sacred. I viewed them with the skills of a teacher of the handicapped. In my attempts to learn more about the disease, I volunteer as a fellow resident to work with my resident friends in group situations.

I group them; not by IQ or age, but by needs. When you read this book, you will see how diverse they are. I hope it gives you some insight into your, your parent, relative's or friend's journey through their experience with the disease. Mine was unpleasant at times, difficult, but also surprisingly good, believe it or not.

Donald Bowling

# CHAPTER 1

## A Gigantic Snake

A gigantic snake covered with ancient Egyptian hieroglyphics slithers past me in my daughter's back yard. A jagged shriek bangs into my left ear and I yell for Melodie, "Come and see!" She sticks her head out of the window and says, "What's happening Dad?" "Look at the size of this snake, it's at least thirty feet long and a foot wide!" "Dad, I only see the garden hose. Are you okay?"

I grab my left ear and think I don't feel okay. "What in the world is wrong with me?" I was a school principal in a state hospital. Now I feel I only have shit for brains. My work in state hospitals had told me about hallucinations. They were only real to the persons who had seen them.

Also, my memory is weird. I don't remember anything about November of last year to March of this year. Melodie told me something about Christmas dinner with my brother Bill. She even showed me a photo of us at the Christmas tree. I do not remember, "What's the matter with me?" They say that you should expect changes to your body after you are eighty, but this is spooky!

Melodie talks me into coming inside and napping. I can't go to sleep. I keep thinking about a hallucinating patient in one state hospital who was pleasant enough, but pleasant enough to kill his mother! Every time I saw him, he was talking to the ceiling, talking to something that I didn't see. He called it God. Unfortunately, One day on a home visit God must have told him to kill his mother. I had to testify in court that he hallucinated about God and a Psychiatrist testified that some "God-talkers" say that God tells them to kill someone. I went to sleep praying for the mother and her boy. Luckily, I only saw a snake that was not there.

I wake up about 8:00 PM and wonder if I have Alzheimer's? Patients in state hospitals don't show this brain disease because their mental illnesses cover over Alzheimer's symptoms and demand chemical medication. I'm familiar with the disease but have never seen patients strongly affected by it.

I *Google* searched on my computer, memory loss and dementia trying to get more information. I found out long-term memory recall is supposed to grow stronger and short term, is not going to work as well. Yes, it is getting like that for me. Like it was yesterday, I can remember in third grade, sticking a girl's hair braid, into my inkwell. I remember her tears and the teacher marching me to the Principal's for a spanking. However, it was only yesterday that I met a beautiful lady whom I cannot recall her name.

Recently, some of the more frustrating events were finding where I parked my car or put my keys. That's no longer a problem because I gave my keys to my daughter and asked her to sell the car. I don't want to be surprised if that giant snake shows up in the crosswalk and I hit someone. My friend and doctor tells me that we all lose our keys sometimes. However, if you don't know what keys are for, you may have Alzheimer's. Have I joined the club? Have I flown over the cuckoo's nest? With that I wet my bed.

# CHAPTER 2

## It's Alzheimer's!

Embarrassment. The most embarrassing moment in my life was being caught at fifteen in the bathroom masturbating. Now it seems I have another to add to the list. How would I admit to my daughter that I just wet my bed? Her presenting me with a chamber pot that she had received from a disgruntled plumber gave us both a needed laugh. Ah, what a wonderful daughter.

I got over my poor attitude in time to hear that we have an appointment with a Neurologist Physician to diagnose my curse. We drove down to her office reviewing what we are going say. We agree to tell her everything.

Melodie tells me to tell the doctor at least three things that she describes to me in lurid detail. After I recover from the shock of what I did, I pinched myself to see if I am awake. I will tell the doctor that I had dressed in one of my best suits at 4:00

AM and woke Melodie up asking her to take me to a meeting in Chicago. Another day I walked down the street without my pants on. One night she found me sitting in a chair in the front room with a bare bottom. I told her that I was just airing out my penis for a little while.

The doctor's office is filled with sleepy people over sixty years of age. The receptionist welcomes us with a smile. We are just in time to see the doctor. We entered the office and saw a very young lady. I tell her about my three sins. She writes a few things and proceeds to give me some oral tests. The doctor tests me for being able to recall five and six place numbers forward and backwards. She shows pictures of men and women and asks me to recall their names by just looking at the pictures without name labels. She asks me all about my sleeping habits and any physical problems I may have.

After about an hour of questions and tests she says, "I think you may have a beginning case of Alzheimer's. I want you to go to the hospital for a brain scan. I'll make an appointment for you." Melodie says that my insurance will pay for most of the test.

Several days later we drive to the hospital for the test. My long-term memory kicks in and I am remembering my last major experience driving to the hospital that opened an old painful memory. Nineteen years ago I followed the ambulance in my car. My wife, Penny, had had a series of treatments on her cancerous pituitary gland and had reached the lowest possible survival level. I cried and prayed that she would recover. I recalled that I had verbally chewed out a truck driver who got between the ambulance and me on the way to the hospital. He gave me the finger and drove past the ambulance in a dangerous fashion. I swear if I'd had a gun, I would have shot at him.

That was then and today is now. We arrived at the section of the hospital with the scanning machines. The scanners looked a lot different than the machines a long time ago and they are quieter. I dress in a hospital gown and wonder why I have to wear a gown that shows my butt. Carefully I get on the table and insert my head in the machine for the brain scan while my bare butt chills on the table. Oh well, why fight the system? The scanner makes a lot of clacking sounds and finally I am shown the dressing room. I can't forget the memories of Penny's death.

We return home that evening for dinner in the backyard. Thankfully, I don't find any traces of the giant snake. I would like to have a barbequed snake, but the garden hose doesn't entice me enough. Instead, we barbecue a section of spare ribs.

The phone rings and the doctor tell us the news that it looks like Alzheimer's. I am glad it isn't cancer. Melodie tells her husband, Cory, that I had done a good job of answering the doctor's questions. Cory says with a smile, "Did you tell her about airing out your penis?" I said, "Sure", with a catch in my throat.

Melodie and Cory ask me what do I want to do? I say, "Find me a place where they can protect me from myself and stop jeopardizing your teaching jobs by taking care of me." Melodie says, "Don't worry about that, but we do have to keep working during the day. I don't think we can afford to have full-time home care. If we find a place that could help you, taxes would not be a problem." Cory says, "I will do your taxes and home care would be difficult." Cory is good at taxes and I trust him completely.

Melodie, Cory and their sons, start looking at Napa's senior facilities. They spend three days checking out places and describe to me a favorite.

I said, "I'm going to my room to read a book called, *The Alzheimer's Prevention Program.* I dug it out of my stuff and had wondered at my choice of buying it six months ago at the bookstore. Scanning the book I found some things that are supposed to make the disease less severe and less lengthy.

Dr. Small says that one of the ways to lessen the effect of Alzheimer's is to manage your stress. My past work required me to present reports to the California Senate Budget Committee for the state hospital system. Talk about stress! I recalled managing the stress from that time. I belonged to a group started by the psychic Edgar Cayce, The Association for Research and Enlightenment. Meditation and prayer is the basic action of the group. I needed to go back to that because I had stopped going to church and meditating regularly in 2008. That was when, Ethel, my second wife had died and I was half mad at God about it.

My kind of meditation started in the Edgar Cayce Bible study group I joined after Evelyn died in 1995. The weekly meeting usually ended with a meditation for about fifteen minutes. It contained a statement of affirmation and prayer for the people in need. Cayce's only formula for meditating developed from his psychic Akashic records, which were action-oriented. The affirmation focused the group on statements like; "God be merciful to me! Help thou my unbelief! Let me see in Him that thou would have me see in my fellow man. Let me see in my brother that I see in Him whom I worship." 262-11* or

"Let virtue and understanding be in me, for my defense is in thee, O Lord, my redeemer, for thou hearest the prayer of the upright in heart." 262-17, A-14 or

"How gracious is thy presence in the earth, O Lord! Be thou the guide, that we, with patience, may run the race which is set before us looking to thee, the Author, the giver of light." 262.24

*Cayce defines prayer and meditation in his book, *A Search for God*, from which I quote and define the numbered section.

## Introduction to Meditation

In this material world we are conscious of the phenomenon of growth. We should be equally aware of spiritual progression that includes both a broadening of understanding of the relationship between the creator and ourselves, and a definite improvement in capabilities to more useful lives. Too much stress has been placed upon the desirability of escaping from physical existence. The average individual has come to look upon spiritual things as being intangible and ethereal, unconnected with normal life.

The eternal question that runs through life; "What was truly valuable in thought, adversity, and experience?" Only from within can come a stable estimate of what is worthwhile. This sense of appreciation of this inner realization is based fundamentally upon an understanding of yourself in relationship to others and yourself in relationship to God. Meditation can be the means to this end.

*(Bible quote from Luke 18:10-14 not shown)*

Prayer and Meditation defined and illustrated

Some individuals give little thoughts to either prayer or meditation. They are satisfied to drift in the current hoping that somehow or somewhere conditions will work out for the best. There are others who seek a better way searching for that light which renews hope and justifies the course of life that is being pursued. Prayer is the concerted effort of our physical consciousness to become attuned to the consciousness of the Creator. It is the attunement of our conscious minds to the spiritual that manifests in a material world. It may be a cooperative experience of many individuals, coming together with one accord and with one mind. Prayer is the pouring out of personality for outward show, to be seen by men (and women.) To others, it means entering unto the closet of the inner self and pouring out the ego so that the inner being may be filled with the spirit of the Father.

## Meditation defined

Meditation is the emptying of ourselves of all that hinders the creative force from rising along the natural channels of our physical bodies to be disseminated through the sensitive spiritual centers in our physical bodies. When meditation is properly entered into, we are made stronger mentally and physically. "He went in the strength of this meat received for many days."(281-13)

Meditation is not musing or daydreaming, but attuning our mental and physical bodies to their spiritual source. It is arousing the mental and spiritual attributes to an expression of their relationship with their Maker. This is true meditation.

Meditation is prayer from within the innerself and partakes not only of the inner physical man (and woman) but also of the soul aroused by the spirit from within. In prayer we speak to God, in meditation God speaks to us."

I now realize that it was really a mistake to stop meditating and worshiping God.

# CHAPTER 3

## I find a real home.

I keep seeing more scary and exciting events as we wait for the admission day. I see a large group of Mexican-American grape pickers in the field next door. They look like Pancho Villa's Guerilla Army to me. I warn Cory and he says, "Don't worry they are just grape pickers."

I worry, first a snake and now a revolution. My God, how bad is this going to be? Will I see the leader of Mexico, President Benito Juarez or Dictator Benito Mussolini of Italy? I think I better go to Aegis and start taking the Namenda pills that my doctor prescribed.

Melodie and Cory take me to the Aegis senior facility on Redwood Road. The building is a beautiful two-story, large home that flies the American and California state flag near the front door. The lobby entrance is very pleasant and a beautiful blond lady, Paula, greets us with a smile. She dials a number on her telephone and a pleasant man named Paul comes and talks to Melodie and Cory about me while Paula asks me about what I like to eat? Paula also asks," Would you like to see a movie at six o'clock this evening?"

Paul took me through a one-way security door and introduced me to Mario. Mario took my suitcase and me to a small room with a bed and said, "This is your temporary room. We will get you a larger room for your bed and the things that you need."

Some elderly ladies walk by and I say to myself, "there are lots of ladies here." I feel good about how I can get along with ladies from the experiences with my two wives.

I married two wonderful women, but not at the same time. They each convinced me that women are the best gender. When I was married to Penny our joint decisions always worked. When I made a decision on my own without Penny or Ethel it only had a chance of working about fifty percent of the time.

At the age of 70, Ethel and I had a great marriage for three years before she died of cancer. I was so pissed off at God that I didn't know what to do. It was like the sick joke; A group of handicapped people going down the street crying, "Why me God, Why me?" A booming voice comes from the sky and says, "IT'S BECAUSE I DON'T LIKE YOU!"

I asked my old friend who is a psychic, "what should I do?" She told me that she had good news for me, " Penny and Ethel have met in heaven and become friends. They are now watching you and laughing at all the mistakes you are making."

I swear from that moment, I sometimes felt their help when I was writing my books. I was using words that weren't even in my vocabulary. When I heard thunder, I knew they were laughing at my mistakes. That made me thank God for big favors. Does that sound crazy? Remember I have Alzheimer's.

Mario takes me into the dining area that has a number of wooden tables and nice chairs set for lunch. He tells me that lunch will be served in ten minutes. I wonder how formal the meals are and he speaks of meals that are just like home. This is going to be your home.

Cordial and patient young ladies served lunch, noise was kept to a minimum and the ladies have to help four or five residents to eat on a one-to-one basis. These ladies were well trained in the "best friend" technique of communicating with residents. The "best friend" theory works when you let your best friend get away with a few weird behaviors because she or he is your best friend. She's careful about using phrases that make you feel more comfortable like, "Need to go to the bathroom?" instead of, "Want to go to the toilet?" Elderly ladies or gentlemen are concerned about kinds of language about personal habits.

Mealtime is when pills are dispensed. A place that cares for folks of 70, 80, or 90 years of age needs to have a system that gets the 20, 30, or 40 correct pills to their residents. Did I say pills? It's a lot. The Aegis system is extremely effective by having their staff deliver them mostly under the supervision of their nurses.

I was interested in watching the variety of eating skills of my friends in the memory unit. One fellow was excellent in his conversational social skills but was only able to feed himself food with his hands, no utensils. He carefully wiped his mouth with the edge of the tablecloth and dropped the napkin on the floor. One woman had the skills of etiquette par excellence and was very critical of her male friend's manners. He, in turn, was very angry about her criticisms.

A young blond lady named Ingrid came during lunch and helped the staff with the one-to-one feeding and then helped them go into the next room that had a number of reclining chairs. Ingrid started by greeting the group and moving people into the semi-circle. About eight of the residents were in wheelchairs and the some were settled in the reclining chairs. They needed their legs to be elevated.

Ingrid starts leading the singing," Coming Round The Mountain," and encouraging them clap their hands to exercise their arms. She continues upper body exercises and sings old favorites like, *Alexander's Ragtime Band, Beer Barrel Polka, Chattanooga Choo Choo, and How much is that doggie (ostrich, kitty, mouse, zebra or elephant) in the window?* She is very creative. She and the group laughs when someone sings "woof, woof!" She joyfully speeds ahead for 30 minutes of fun exercising, and ends with an art lesson using watercolors.

She likes to play the role of 'smile therapist'. Many years of troubled existence has frozen some resident's faces into frowns. Ingrid melts those frowns into smiles by singing, "Smile, Though Your Heart is Aching." She also physically moves their lips to a smile.

I immediately fall in love with her and ask her to marry me. She tells me she has a boyfriend. I think about my quick marriage maneuver. Did I get her positive attention? I probably should know the lady if I'm going to ask that question. Will she ever speak to me again? I'm like her grandfather. Ingrid reminds me of my late wife Penny and I feel I would like to lead groups in singing and ball games like she does. Later I ask Paul if I could volunteer for an hour or two a day in leading games and singing like I did with patients in state hospitals. He approves if I would work under the supervision of Ingrid. That is great!

Another one of Ingrid's crowning achievements is her monthly schedule of, 'Life's Neighborhood events and Activities'.

Each month's events show residents in what they can participate with the leadership of activity directors; Ingrid, Mindy and Nancy and two volunteer assistants; Lucille, a talented singer and me, Don, a retired school principal, who are residents. Also staff; Holly's daughter, Lisbeth, works with groups in music appreciation when she can.

## Here is an excerpt from Ingrid's calendar; 8/13

- 9:00 Current events, newspaper's news and horoscope, are read by Don.

- 9:30 Green ball bounce; kick and bat indoors ballgame by Nancy and Don

- 10:00 Smoothies break, frozen health drink by Ingrid, Nancy and Mindy

- 10:30 Balance fit; balance exercises to prevent falling also by Ingrid, Nancy and Mindy

- 10:45 Picture bingo developed by Ingrid

- 1:00 Walk, roll or relax with Nancy, Ingrid and Mindy

- 1:30 Masterpiece art by Ingrid, Nancy and Mindy with collage, coloring or crafts

- 3:00 Don's book club

- 4:00 Oktoberfest party for everybody

Activities are an all inclusive description of work performed by rehabilitation therapists. This setting with its diverse clientele requires quick-witted, adaptable persons.

I begin to feel that I am getting clear of my dementia. Then I am startled to see the light fixture above my bed moving, so not quite clear yet.

# CHAPTER 4

## My friends changed personalities.

I call my unit of 20 friends "The Memory Place." We all have our memory problems. I cannot remember Christmas dinner with my brother in the middle last year's tremendous memory hole. I don't remember many important experiences because of my dementia. I forgot many things from when I was young in school and with my parents. I also forgot things about my own family, my marriages and my jobs.

I was taught at UCLA, as a teacher, that we are a product of our experiences. If Alzheimer's causes damage throughout our brain by a random, "crap-shoot" of plaques and tangle deposits, then our personalities change completely after that disease. My friends in memory care are changed by dementia at old age. Their new personalities are a random arrangement of lost memories; they are like snowflakes, no two are alike.

Several years ago, my friend, Jeb, moved into assisted care with his wife. She died last year. He is kind of a mute person who wanders around either fully clothed or nude. He has grown into a stubborn fellow with short responses like, "How about that?" or "Sure, good!" I praised him when he stood up in a song and exercising session and danced to the rhythm of the song. His son told me he had been a successful executive. Presently, his personality is a product of his old age and Alzheimer's dementia. Friends, relatives and family mostly remember Jeb as a successful executive, not the person that I like now.

The staff here focuses on good memories and exercises of any kind that will strengthen the ability to recall. Ingrid incorporates memory exercises for the group by having them call-out the months of the year, forward and backwards during exercising and days of the week in that same manner.

I can't look at my resident friend's medical records, but when I can, I ask their visiting relatives what these residents did for a living. I get everything from, "I don't know." to, "Thank you for being interested in Nancy."

Here are some of my favorite friends. (Names are changed)

Bob: He has a cheerful personality, exudes social skills with a special skill in social banter. He is physically-able to lead circle ball games and include all players in the game. He is able to develop their kicking, throwing and batting the ball.

According to his son he coached Little League Baseball teams. He also is very friendly with Nancy but refrains from touching her. They laugh and joke a lot. He is very confused in his physical awareness of objects. He is confused in Ingrid's exercises when she calls for motions of the arms or legs; he cannot distinguish between his arms and legs on command.

Nancy: She sits near Bob whenever possible and they have an almost brother/sister relationship. She can speak logically and also help Bob in his coaching role. She seems to get along with everyone. She has good art skills in coloring.

She helps Holly and Becca with their rocky relationship.

Becca: She can swear like a man, sing like a bird and reacts negatively to any command. She likes to chastise other's behaviors like Bob's poor eating skills, which he doesn't appreciate. She quickly swings from angel to a harsh disciplinarian. She speaks well and understands a lot of subtle messages. When I asked the group what kind of clothes do you like? She said none. She asked me publically, do you like sex?

Holly: She's a 99 year's old cutie that only expects the best behavior of 'yours truly'. She reacted sharply to my describing farts and criticized my belief in St. Peter and Heaven. She is a darling person who can always be counted on saying a positive thing or attacking stupid statements. She is always good at coloring and staying in between the lines. I love her.

Helen: She's a stone-faced 96 year's old (add another ten years to my 86 and I might also be stone-faced). Her facial expressions emoted in my teaching groups seemed to say, "I don't know what the hell I'm doing here. Let's get this show on the road." She did not speak or seemingly could not speak.

I begin to use a speech technique used by my late wife, Penny, who was a speech therapist. I started singing an easy song with a group of about twelve 'friends.' We sang, "Home on the Range" and Helen began to mouth the words. When I saw her lips move I couldn't hear a voice, but her lips mouthed the whole song with the other singers. Elated, I asked the group if this was the start of the baseball season? I asked if anyone knew a baseball song? I heard a small voice start singing, "Take me out to the ballgame. Take me out with the crowd."

I heard someone say, "My God, she can sing!" I said, "And she can talk!"

Nancy said, "I share my room with her and I have never heard her say a word." Helen then said, "What the hell are you waiting for? I want to sing the rest of the song!"

Marcy: She can be seen carrying around a life-sized baby doll. She'll talk to it and place it in a crib in her room. Marcy is gentle and kind most of the time. She can speak in a gentle, sweet voice or shout loudly. One time she expressed her undying love for me, and a few minutes later, kicked me in the groin for taking a ball from her. I now consider wearing a sports cup around her and I stopped taking balls from her.

John: He's a handsome 70-year-old favorite of the female staff. He has tremors and needs a great deal of one-on-one care in feeding, dressing, bathing and toileting. He constantly mumbles and talks to someone who is not there. He has Parkinson's as well as Alzheimer's. Communication is difficult with him. Often the other Alzheimer's residents of our memory care group ignore him.

Sophie: She has a noble appearance when she arrives in her wheelchair. She speaks clearly, but incoherently. Her body looks gaunt, like a concentration camp survivor. Her meals are supplemented with a protein drink and a host of pills. She's handled very carefully and is at risk for falling. Her physical abilities are awkward and weak, but she appears to enjoy being included in our activities. She does not seem to be able to make her needs known.

To be fair I will describe myself in the same fashion that I described my fellow residents.

Don: He is a little overweight. His controlled diet has helped him to lose weight. He's around 200 pounds from the 263 pounds he weighed eight months earlier. He wants to live in this place forever and his state pension and social security will pay for it. He's a little awkward in the morning but he makes it to the breakfast table in an upright position. He is known for appreciating the opposite sex but he needs to refrain from asking them to marry him.

## How Do I Help the Alzheimer Friends with which I Live?

I taught the handicapped for 20 years and my first impulse is to develop plans to answer their important, special needs. What about the elderly Alzheimer residences?

How would I work with me? Take my tendency to overeat; stop eating a diet high in carbohydrates and fat. Focus on a complete diet of protein, fruit and vegetables. I am unable to drive because of my side effects from necessary medications and the dementia. That keeps me away from my favorite haunt, Burger King. Perhaps a few sessions with Weight Watchers would be risky, and I might lose my desire to eat, maybe not. My extra 63 pounds might have led me to an early heart attack.

Bob, who is touchy from the criticism of his eating habits by Becca, was scarfing down everything in sight with his hands. It more than likely was because that part of his brain had lost its previous training from childhood. Several short lessons on how to use a fork, spoon and knife in a cooking class of his favorite food would lead to better eating skills and don't forget his favorite food. It would be the purpose and reward of the lesson.

I'm might be a maniac about grouping students, but that was my main career skill in setting up a program. If possible, get a majority of people with the same need.

The cooking of favorite food works wonders with training retarded children and brain-damaged adults.

I realize that I am simplifying a very complex transition because of Alzheimer's and old age. However, I just want to make it clear that you must be aware of the fact that you are trying to help change a loved one that is now very different. There will be a lot of buttons that will not work. However you can create new ways to solve their needs. Remember, you sometimes have to teach a human by having them successfully repeat an action correctly, sometimes eleven times in a row.

Grouping these friends was necessary. Three of the women have emotional switches that can make them angels or devils. Four of my friends had physical handicaps, and I don't take the ball away from anybody.

I had to be ready to assist them for the bathroom on a regular basis. A staff member would take the ladies to the bathroom. My experience with the men consisted of leading some to the toilet, helping them unzip their pants and moving aside when the stream flowed. Others went into the bathroom, closed the door, washed their hands and left. Some had to be reminded to perform that sanitary exercise. One man urinated on my door to show his disdain at one of my actions during the day. My fan club did not include him.

A modified indoor kick ball game gave them exercise and coordination development while seated in a circle of chairs. I gave Bob the job of player-coach and Nancy, his assistant. Bob could see who needed help with kicking or whacking. My job is toileting, rewarding good plays and chasing the big green ball with my walker. Helen of course was in charge of heckling. I was fascinated by their endurance in these games. One game lasted one hour before the group wanted to rest.

I assisted Nancy or my dream girl, Ingrid, in art activities that were very creative and allowed my friends to have successful experiences in creativity. Collage meant searching through a lot of old magazines and looking for happy people. When the figures were cut out they were pasted in some kind of design on construction paper. Each person shared their creation to the oohs and ahhs of the group.

Another exercise was called blind drawing. Everyone was given a yellow crayon and told to close their eyes. White squares of paper were taped to their tables and they were asked to scribble all around the paper for 30 seconds. Then they opened their eyes and were given a box of crayons and asked to color in the white areas between the yellow lines. Twelve colorful stained glass church windows were put up on the bulletin board again to the oohs and ahhs of everyone.

Ingrid has a special kind of Bingo game; it has heads of animals instead of numbers. When 'B' owl is called, a poker chip covers the picture of the owl. Bingo winners get a chocolate kiss and no other kisses grow from this success. This game is second only to dinnertime.

# CHAPTER 5

## This is home sweet home?

I meet a jolly fellow that seemingly looks of a "Good Ole Boy". He is pleasant to be around and knows how to get involved with lots of staff and fifty residents. His name is Dobby and his laughter can be heard all over the lobby and starts my day with a smile. Ethel is a lady who will dance alone beautifully when the right music is in the air. She leads a clique of four or five ladies in her activities. Dobby and Ethel are aware of each other but that's all. They and their friends provide a social dynamo to this very select society in which I live.

Friday afternoon is fun, live musician performers and we have drinks with just a tiny bit of alcohol. A plethora of musicians and singers are available from the Napa Valley to entertain the residents. A twenty-year-old guitarist and singer swing the moods of the residents to snap their fingers and sway to the music of rock and roll. Several members of the audience are moved to sing along or get up and dance a solo fandango.

An 87 and 93 year-old married couple plays piano, guitar and violin together. A few squawks and squeals from the violin's strings fail to dampen the audience's mood. Everyone is impressed!

A daring older man on a flying piano from Broadway's 1920's thrills everyone with his unending memory of lyrics of yesterday and grinds the bones of the old audience. This mature genius of the keyboard sends everybody singing to the dining room. Ingrid, Mindy and Nancy score again with a hit.

Lots of games are scheduled everyday to keep people active and exercised. We have dominos, picture bingo, Uno, puzzles and sorting, war, sand sculptures and a number of verbal games and jokes. In this setting, during the first months of my Alzheimer soaked tenure, I stumbled from one almost conscious memory to another.

My large office/bedroom was decorated with photographs of my family, wives and friends. This is a pleasant tradition of the facility to make me feel at home. My iMac computer, printer, flat screen television, chairs and bed all add up to a great space for me. However, I had to first learn again operating the computer, printer and television. It was startling for my friends to see my first emails!

I have has some sort of hallucinations about this set up. In exploring this large apartment-like building I mistakenly see other replicates. How kind of the facility to give me two other working/sleeping places. When I looked outside in these daydreams, I saw two buildings instead of the one in which I was living. These strange daydreams survived my "memory hole."

What was I seeing? Was it old age or Alzheimer's? If you or your loved ones have this sort of hallucinations, look out!

Appropriately, the Namenda pills started to "kick-in" on April Fools Day. While the big memory hole blotted out the previous months of November, December, January, February and March. In April, I received the gift of life again.

My daughter and her family, and the great staff kept mum about my weird and painful experiences during this period. I probably would have walked into the Pacific Ocean if I had known of my behavior. It took me another three months to almost completely shake out the clumps of protein in brain's neurons and the dementia out of my body as well.

In July, I started to work with my groups in singing, sports and exercising. I got into the groove of helping Bob, Nancy, Becca, Holly, Helen, Marcy, Jeb, Sophia and others. I saw it helped them climb out of their memory holes. It also helped me a to meet new friends, crawl out of my hole, and start to feel good. I slept all night instead of the two or three hours I had slept intervened with listening to music.

I was doing fine until my daughter let it slip that she had kept a journal on me during the big hole in my life.

# CHAPTER 6

## I Get "Brownie Points."

I wake up one morning after dreaming about ladies. I was mainly admiring them, they were charming, talkative, thin, plump, gorgeous, and most of all perfect. I would not know what Edgar Cayce would say about the meaning of my dream. For an 86-year-old male it certainly wasn't a wet one.

All I knew was it was about the gender that I feel should rule the world. Here I am, in a place where ninety percent of the individuals are women. I am smitten with women- old, young, tall, short, medium, tan, brown, black and yellow. I am living with older versions of the sex praised by H. Allen Smith in his magical philosophic book that showed a day that either the world was all made up of women or men. With women in charge he saw world peace, and progress in all areas. In a world populated by men, constant warfare, greed and factories turning out millions of female robots as sex toys, cursed it. Many REAL ladies surround me!

My two wives had convinced me, in my two marriages, that females are superior. Penny had convinced me that sexual chromosomes were the major clue. I remember that women have X chromosomes and men have Y ones. What's a Y but an X with a leg missing? So our missing leg disables us. Had enough? Women often live longer are smarter and delightful.

I was pretty despondent after the death of my two wives. I told you how a psychic helped me the first time by saying my wives had met each other after their deaths. Helen released me from my depression by telling me that they were still with me. This psychic woman had worked for the FBI and the CIA. I think she had great intelligence by telling me that they were watching and would help me. I liked that better than the story that they were laughing at me.

A bi-monthly complaints meeting is held at my care home with a committee of a ratio of one man to ten women. I attended one of their meetings which a woman discussed human rights and the cost of services. One male had a very important complaint "Do not serve rocky road ice cream at the dining room." "Wow, how macho!"

One night, after dark, I wanted to go outside to mail a letter. I'm sure I knew that we have a pickup box. Alzheimer's had a creepy way of acting after dark. I know that I should know that you don't leave a place like Aegis after dark. I walked for about a mile looking for a post office. I was walking in the gutter of a very busy street when a red light started flashing from a Highway Patrol car. He asked me where I lived. I told him I lived at Aegis. He said," Can I take you home, Sir?" "Sure", I said. When we got to Aegis, he talked to the manager while I sat in the lobby. I found myself being followed everywhere I went for three weeks. I guess I earned the title of 'escape risk'. I did not like the notoriety and the problems it caused. It's a case of Alzheimer's poor judgment.

I continued my volunteering with the memory unit. It must have earned me some 'brownie points.' Paul and Ingrid gave me a nametag to wear, like a real employee. I was invited to attend a special day at the Oakland A's Baseball stadium for a special Aegis employee day.

According to Ingrid, this was going to be a traditional employee benefits day for those staff who could be spared from duties at the five Aegis senior facilities around the San Francisco Bay area. We started planning for a skit in competition with the other four facilities.

Ingrid creatively designed a funny play that would have me being escorted into the scene by six serious, security persons. I would escape and Booga Looga to a rap song sung by one of our chefs. Ingrid's creativity won the Napa's entry for the coveted trophy to shine in our lobby for the next year.

A great barbecue fed the hundred plus group, with a raffle of a couple of TV's and other electronic prizes were won. The Seattle manager spoke to the employees with gratitude. The

Oakland A's won the game with Huston. The vigor of Ingrid with a baseball mitt was inspiring even if she failed to get a foul ball in the forth inning.

This sort of company treat shows part of the reason for their employee loyalty. I am beginning to enjoy the benefits of being a non-paid volunteer resident. My disease still appears to be going towards remission, and I get lots of praise.

I get allowed to eat in the resident's dining when I want to get away from the family-style dining of the memory unit.

# CHAPTER 7

## The five-month silver memory hole.

I have finally given up on my search for the mythical room-replicates. My hallucinating has stopped except for a little movement of my light fixture after a hard workday. I think that is going to be my loadstone for seeing if my physician can declare me in remission.

I wake up after a good night's sleep. I feel like I am in remission and I want to celebrate. So I called Melodie and tell her. She asks if the doctor has given me that information. I say, sheepishly, "Well no, but I feel great." She says, "Your birthday is coming up soon and I feel like we should celebrate with some sort of party."

She and I decide to get together at her house and plan a party. She picks me up and takes me to her house. Once home, she decided to also pick up a fellow teacher and bring her to help us plan. When she leaves to pick up her friend I settle down in her kitchen to find a snack. I spotted her journal and decided to take it home to read. I'll regret what I found out about what I did.

## Melodie's Journal

November 10th, Dad tells me that he saw lots of people getting into his car.

15th, Dad came over at 8:00 PM thinking it was morning. Is he sun downing? I put a sign up in his room, ONLY GO OUTSIDE WHEN IT IS LIGHT.

December 10, 2:00 AM, Dad is banging on the back door and claiming that the hospital is creating a mess outside his door. He wants to call the police.

11th, Dad came over and reminded me and Cory that we had better start planning on an educational workshop for his teachers and do it quickly or he will get mad.

12th, Dad told us he had a lady visitor at his place and she would be returning soon. He was well dressed and she never showed up.

18th, Dad is having trouble with uncontrolled urination, called hospital for help. Nurse says that urinary tract infections may be the trouble. Go to ER, doctor confirmed UTI and felt he had Lewy Bodies dementia. Later it was confirmed that his kidneys were in trouble from medication misuse. Dad fell in the bathroom, did not hit his head. This troubled day continues and Cory and I are weak from it.

We went to ER again. Further examination and testing led to Dad's admission to the hospital. I stayed with him as much as possible. Dad started sun downing and trying to get up many times during the night. Nurses were amazingly patient. Dad was very negative and upset a lot. I was not able to get the hospital to give him antidepressants. The discharge nurse advocated for him to go into assisted living. The family and I looked at facilities and decided that the Springs was the best. The staff were so understanding of his behavior.

24th, Dad's catheter became another pain for him. A nurse was provided to mainly assist him with that appliance.

29th, Yeah! The catheter is removed.

31st, Dad began to sundown again. Conducted inappropriate conversations with women, and entered other private apartments.

January 5th, Diagnosed with UTI again and admitted in hospital. He had anxiety, inappropriate language, hallucinations and no sleeping.

8th, He's angry, with belligerent refusal to go to the doctor's. Only goes when nurse will accompany him. Constant falling asleep, coughing, and confusion. Getting antibiotics, inhaler and chest x-ray.

9th, It's the same confusion, thinks he's at hospital, instead of the Springs. 10th, He's still keeping his chin down with shallow breathing, hallucinating, falls asleep while eating and has difficulty communicating and no sleeping. Since this began, he has been calling out throughout the night. Worries that he needs to talk to his lawyer about his situation. Needs reassurance that the Springs has no control of his money. Continues to need 24-hour hour supervision. He wanders constantly getting up without knowing where he is going. He needs help eating because of his sleeping problems and only sleeps an hour for every twelve hours at night.

11th, He has an ER request for a doctor. He is a tiny bit more lucid, walking with a walker and sleeping a little more.

12th, Hospitalized with catheter and needs more medication.

January 13th, keeping him in hospital to check on medications.

14th, Hospital wants to move Dad to skilled nursing facility. Instead we had Aegis evaluate him but he is discharged to Springs because a Springs' nurse recommends continuing with 24 hour nursing care. Needs have increased significantly. Has catheter. Dr. wants to try Seroquel but it turns out to exacerbate hallucinations and oppositional behavior.

15th, Appointment with urologist because of urine retention and enlarged prostate. May always need catheterization. Two days later he still has that problem, Dr. continues catheter, Dad later pulls it off and was taken to ER to reinsert.

16th, Cory and I meet with staff of Springs about Aegis Senior Facility. That night, Dad strips and wants to go outside of room. Health aid tells him to put some clothes on. He pulls her hair and she gives sleeping pill to him.

20th, Catheter out.

23rd, Neurology apt. verbal testing and history taken. Did very poorly, spoke inappropriately and hallucinated.

25th, Moved dad to Aegis facility. He is happy with their nice lunch. He called me at 8:00 PM and asked why he was there.

26th, Called Maureen the nurse at Aegis about his edema at his ankles. Ordered compression stockings.

27th, Took his autoharp to him so he could sing songs. Played piano with him singing, "You are my Sunshine." We talked about mom's attempts to use an experimental drug for Cushing's Syndrome before she died. Dad has not sun downed for two weeks.

29th, Urology checkup. Doctor finds retaining at 250 cc and a blockage of Prostate. Recommends green light surgery.

30th, Dad pulled out catheter and doctor switched to one with large bulb on end to stay in bladder.

31st, Dad shows unhappiness with Aegis staff then expresses his love for them.

February 2nd, No sun downing and not fiddling with catheter.

4th, Difficult night, needed lots of attention. Nurse removed catheter, urologist says okay before surgery.

5th, Green light surgery. Picked Dad up at 7:15. Dad is fine after green light. Took him to Aegis at 2:00 PM. We got meds at drugstore.

Got a phone call from Aegis saying Dad wanted to commit suicide. Gave him a pep talk. Aegis gives him meds for sleeping.

10th, Dad is sun downing again. He is having trouble using the phone. Also he is unplugging lights, television, and the computer. He has trouble keeping track of cash I gave him. Most of it ends up in trash. Aegis staff returns it to me.

14th, Dad's talking of suicide, again.

15th, Dad is enjoying funny videos with peers. Great mood. I ate lunch with him and he talked about how he feels that he is responsible for his moods. He says he wants me to remind him of this when he is in a bad mood.

18th, Dad is having difficulty with handwriting. He hasn't been able to use his computer since November. He showed no interest in my showing him how to send emails. He keeps falling asleep during meals and other activities. Dad carries on inappropriate sexual conversations with himself.

March 7th, He is having massive internal bleeding from his UTI, son David is here from Saint Louis and takes him to ER. Hospital admits him and catheterizes him. The hospital runs many bags of saline solution to heal bladder and eliminate blood. He's in the hospital days for the saline treatment. He has trouble at night and tries to wander. Finally urine is clear and catheter is removed. He is still not holding his head up.

21st, Aegis calls and says that Dad is straining to breath. They intubate him because he can't breath. He goes to ICU for a few days before they can remove breathing tube. They have found that a piece of hard candy was lodged in his airway. He has become very angry.

22nd, (Dad remembers this episode, this the end of the memory hole.) Aegis reports to me that Dad has left in the middle of the night and walked to a nearby 7-ll store. Police return him. Aegis moves him to memory care unit for his safety. He is very angry with me.

March, He is moved to his present room and is very happy.

May 1st, Dad gets a PET scan that shows his brain's Alzheimer-like damage. The neurologist prescribes Namenda and he shows great improvement after one month.

June 10th, The sun downing is gone and he begins to use his computer and phone again. He can read effectively and begins to help teach his peers in the memory unit in reading, singing and exercising. He is protected from leaving the unit. Dad develops a book club and becomes a resident who can go out to city restaurants for lunch on Fridays. He chooses to stay in memory care with his friends who need help. He then decides to write a book about his journey through Alzheimer's.

# CHAPTER EIGHT

## What makes the memory hole, silver?

I shake my head when I read Melodies' notes. What a whirlwind of events. I am very thankful that I didn't steal the journal until June. That's when I started to stick my head up out of the hole of dementia. I'm sure it could have made me fall back into the hole.

When I admitted that I had stolen it, my daughter said, "I didn't tell you the worst part of your escapade." That was my punishment for stealing it. What had I done? I'm sure it was sexual. Did I have sex with a Kangaroo? No, I don't even hop well.

I guess I will have to carry that to my grave. What's worse than what I had already done? Just to tally up the bad news from dementia and old age, I feel that I am emotionally capable of knowing what happened in my memory hole from November 2014 to March 2015.

Where do I get the silver lining? The memory block saved me from suicide. Think of the times referenced in Melodies' Journal, "I want to kill myself." So, it's a memory hole with a silver lining, "I'm still alive." After reading the journal, I discovered how sick and obnoxiously badly I behaved. I had pulled the nurses hair and even talked dirty to them. The memory barrier saved my sanity of the embarrassment.

The urinary tract infection could have been caused by poor comprehension of sanitary needs, the prostate or old age. I am now drinking lots of cranberry juice. I still don't like catheters with their impositions and tubing. However, I remain thankful for their preservation of my health.

My sun downing only bothered me when I went to breakfast and found out it was dinner. I first found out about this condition when I was in college. I worked graveyard shift in an oil field. It sometimes led me to waking up after an hour of daytime sleep, thinking it was time to go back to work. Sun downing led to me being fired when I reported to work at 9:00 AM a number of times.

Many trips to the ER and hospital may have become tiresome to people, the two care facilities, and my family. I am sure it was tiresome with my pulling out cords from catheters and machines for fluids and air. In general, I may not have made it during those almost 5 months of my memory hole if it hadn't been for all those wonderful people who helped me. Now I can put my behavior problems, poor sanitation and psychotic actions behind me.

## What do we do now?

I wrote this book to give positive direction for people interested in or fearful of getting dementias. Some of my life I have been a part-time health enthusiast. If you read the story of my life at the end of this book, you will see I flip-flopped whenever there were crises. The sickness and deaths of my two wives Penny and Ethel were terrible crises. The conflict in Korea that lead to my being drafted into the Army was extremely heart wrenching at times. Each crisis could be a blow to some healthy habits, and possibly cause depression. Some of my healthy habits were; exercise, eating right, going to church, meditation and spending quality time with friends and family.

Remember the real estate saying? It's location, location, and location. In the case of getting this disease, it's time, time, time and some genetics. Consider the importance of time for being vulnerable to the collection of plaques and tangles in parts of the brain. When did they start? How can we verify that enough have collected at key points to kill the brain cells? The PET brain scan is the only way doctors can tell. Strange behaviors and losing the keys don't tell us. Maybe someday we can stop the plaque and tangles from accumulating, but not now. Drugs like Namenda stopped my damage from the protein nodes of the Lewy Bodies.

Take my experience; I made it to 85 until my Alzheimer's showed up. With my haphazard self-care I was really lucky. I was able to get to treatment by a lifesaving daughter who made the right decisions for me.

Besides the time element we have to remember my 'snow-flake' experience that no two Alzheimer patients are alike. The random accumulation of proteins nodes in the brain will result in chaos of symptoms in Lewy Bodies. What worked for me, may not work for you, your relative, or friend. So treatment has to be a shotgun (or broad) approach to relieving the diseased person.

## What is the broad approach?

I continue to 'break sweat' exercise for an hour a day. It's not easy because of my arthritic legs. I push my walker up and down the carpeted hallways at a brisk walk. I'm known as Dangerous Don McGrew to my friends and staff. I exercise my upper body with boxing exercises I learned at UCLA with 5 pound weights on my wrists for about 20 or 30 minutes. I'm not called Rocky but I get a lot of eye-rolling from my friends and staff. Our social life and activiities seem to fit Dr. Small's suggestions as well as our meals.

Part-time meditating and good health practices held off disease and confirms to me that Dr. Small's prescriptions for prevention works. My approach would group people by age and symptoms. Grouping people who are 50 years old and have no symptoms I would suggest reading Dr. Small's *The Alzhei-mer's Prevention Program*. I would also suggest that they follow his program for the rest of their lives.

Those who have been diagnosed positive by a PET brain scan should read his book if possible and have their caregivers read it to learn about lessening the severity of dementia.

Wait, who is this fellow who thinks he knows all about the disease? I am a teacher, have the disease and I read the prevention book. I am better and I lessened the severity of its craziness by following Dr. Small's program. Also I wanted to share with you my experiences in memory care, and what helped me and my friends.

## The Myths, Maybes and Mores About Alzheimer's

Doctor Small MD of the UCLA Longevity Center and his wife, Gigi Vorgan answer questions that the public pose about Alzheimer's dementia. This section is a reprint from their 'New Resources' in the book, *The Alzheimer's Prevention Program.*

*Q:* Is it true that a new drug is being tested as an Alzheimer's disease treatment?

*A:* Yes, so far, the tests have been performed only on mice. Cancer drugs generally work by preventing the growth of abnormal cells. University of Pennsylvania scientists are testing a drug called EpoD (short for epothilone D) that was developed to treat cancer because the compound over stabilizes the tiny tubules necessary for cancer cells to divide and proliferate—meaning the cancer does not grow or increase. Also EpoD can penetrate the brain at relatively low doses that don't cause side effects. The scientists realized that this ability to strengthen microtubules might help vulnerable brain cells in Alzheimer's disease by fortifying the micro tubes that comprise the misfolded proteins of tau tangles in an Alzheimer's brain. The mice the scientists used in their tests had a human Alzheimer's gene, which impaired their cognition—the animals tended to get lost when crawling through a maze that should have been familiar.

As predicted, EpoD stopped further brain buildup of tau tangles, and the mice were less forgetful when wandering through their mazes. The drug has not yet been tested in humans nor has it been approved as a cancer treatment so, even though these initial results are promising, it may be years before we know if EpoD will be effective for patients with Alzheimer's dementia or those at risk for developing the disease.

$Q$: I heard that some scientists discovered that Alzheimer's spreads through the brain like an infection. Should I be worried about catching the disease from someone who has it?

$A$: Swedish scientists from Linkoping University reported that toxic proteins are transferred from brain cell to brain cell, but you have no need to worry about being infected by an Alzheimer's disease bug. It is not an infection like a cold or pneumonia but a spread of cellular dysfunction from cell to cell within an effected brain. For many years, scientists have known that the disease spreads through the brain in a characteristic pattern expanding through the cortex, the outer rim of cells that control most mental abilities, but this research was the first time that the process was depicted at the cellular level. In laboratory experiments, the researchers showed that a sick brain cell could "infect" other cells nearby. Because this breakthrough study helps scientists understand how Alzheimer's progresses, it offers an opportunity to develop new treatments to stop the spread of the disease throughout the brain.

$Q$: A coworker told me that diabetes doubles the risk for getting Alzheimer's disease. I've had diabetes for years. Should I be worried about developing Alzheimer's?

$A$: A large scale Japanese study showed that people who had diabetes were twice as likely to develop Alzheimer's disease and had a greater risk for any form of dementia. To confirm the suspected connection between diabetes and dementia, investigators from Kyushu University followed 1,000 volunteers for 15 years. Of the 230 research subjects who developed dementia, those who had diabetes had a 74 percent higher risk of developing dementia either from Alzheimer's, small strokes in the brain, or some other cause. The scientists found that the odds of subjects with diabetes getting Alzheimer's disease was about double compared to the subjects who did not have diabetes.

Precisely how diabetes leads to Alzheimer's and other dementias is not certain—it could result from small strokes in the brain known as micro-vascular changes, decreased blood flow, or inability of brain cells to get enough glucose, which is the primary problem in diabetes. The body becomes resistant to the effects of insulin, the hormone that transports glucose from the blood into cells.

Two of the key Alzheimer's prevention strategies—physical exercise and healthy nutrition—are known to prevent diabetes and improve symptoms of the disease. Getting started and remaining on an Alzheimer's prevention program will help your body fight off diabetes and increase the likelihood that you will stave off symptoms of Alzheimer's disease as well.

*Q:* Is it true that air pollution can speed up mental decline and even increase small strokes in the brain?

*A:* A recent study from Brown University demonstrated an association between short-term exposure to air pollution (at levels considered safe) and an increased risk for a stroke. Long-term exposure was associated with faster cognitive decline. The heightened risk for a stroke occurred within 12 to 14 hours of exposure, and it was associated with pollution from automobile traffic in particular. These findings suggest that avoiding exposure to smog is another way to maintain brain health and avoid cognitive decline.

$Q$: I read somewhere that eating fish can make your brain larger. Is that possible?

$A$: It's true—fish eaters have larger brains, and, in general, a bigger brain is a better brain, especially when volume is preserved in areas controlling cognition. Researchers at the University of Pittsburgh performed MRI brain scans on 260 volunteers who had been followed for 10 years. They found that those who ate fish regularly had less shrinkage in areas of their brains controlling memory compared with volunteers who did not eat much fish. Regular fish eaters also had a lower risk for developing mild cognitive impairment or Alzheimer's disease. The subjects with bigger brains ate fish between one to four times each week.

Scientists are not exactly sure how fish preserves brain size and health, but they describe some interesting theories. The omega-3 fatty acids in fish likely protect the brain from neuronal destruction due to inflammation and oxidation. Omega-3 fats have anti-inflammatory effects that counteract the neuron-destructive brain inflammation that results from aging, being overweight, or avoiding regular exercise. The brain-protective fats also fight oxidative stress that causes wear and tear on our brain cells as we age. Study volunteers who ate fried fish rather than grilled or baked fish had smaller brains and higher risks for memory-decline—this is not surprising since fried fish does not have a high concentration of omega-3 fats.

Fish lovers often worry about eating too much fish, and most authorities recommend eating it only twice a week due to concern about mercury exposure. However, avoiding swordfish, shark, and other large predatory  fish will lower your chances of ingesting too much mercury.  Also, don't forget that tilapia is a fish to skip if you want your omegas-3 benefits.  For people who don't like fish, an omega-3 supplement is a good idea.  I recommend 1,000 milligrams each day, and make sure it contains brain protective docosahexaenoic acid or DHA.

*Q:* I saw on TV that doctors had used electric probes to stimulate the brain and it improved memory and symptoms of Alzheimer's. Is it like electroshock therapy and is it dangerous?

*A:* In a small study of five Alzheimer's patients with mild dementia, electrical stimulators were implanted in brain memory centers. To power the stimulators pacemaker-sized battery packs were implanted under the skins of each patient's chest. After a year, the scientists found that the patient's brain memory centers were functioning better as measured by PET scans, and the brain function improvement correlated with better memory scores.  The findings are encouraging but need to be repeated in a larger group of patients.  Although the patients tolerated the treatment well, scientists are now studying less invasive ways to stimulate these same brain memory centers, through electrodes placed on the scalp, rather than implanted surgically.

*Q:* Everyone is talking about an impending Alzheimer's epidemic.  What's going to happen in the next few decades? Are we going to become a nation of demented Baby boomers?

*A:* In March of 2012, the Alzheimer's Association reported that here in the U.S. we're spending $200 billion each year caring for Alzheimer's victims.  As 80 million U.S. baby boomers start reaching the age of 65, their risk for the disease grows.

By 2050 we can expect more than 100 million Alzheimer patients worldwide if we do nothing to fight the disease.

Another frightening revelation was that one out of every seven Alzheimer's patients lives alone. By definition, patients with dementia cannot take care of themselves and need help from others.

This crisis led President Obama to sign the National Alzheimer's Project Act to accelerate research, education, and care giving efforts. Large-scale drug prevention trials are already underway, but it will take years for these studies to yield results. Scientists at the University of California, San Francisco, have concluded that up to half of Alzheimer's cases are attributable to risk factures under our own control. They estimated that if we could reduce modifiable risk factors (e.g., stop smoking, start exercising lose weight) by 25 percent, we could potentially prevent as many as 500,000 cases of Alzheimer's in the U.S. and 3 million worldwide. While we're waiting for science to catch up, there's no reason not to do everything we can to protect our brain health. An Alzheimer's prevention program will improve your memory ability right away and likely delay the onset of Alzheimer's symptoms in the future.

$Q$: I have been tested and found out I have a genetic risk for Alzheimer's disease. Should I even bother starting a prevention program? I mean, what's the use?

$A$: Having a genetic risk for Alzheimer's disease is no reason to give up on your brain health—genetic factors only account for part of the risk. Scientists at Washington University in St. Louis found that even people with the APOE-4 generic risk for Alzheimer's disease have control over their brain aging.

Only 20 percent of the population who are APO-4 carriers are more likely to get Alzheimer's symptoms at a younger age than non-carriers, but even for them that fate is not is not inevitable, and regular physical exercise may play an important role in an individual's outcome.

During these studies, the investigators performed PET scans that measured the amount of brain amyloid deposits in 201 people, ages 45 to 88. These amyloid protein deposits are associated with Alzheimer's disease symptoms. Volunteers with an active lifestyle had significantly less brain amyloid deposits compared with those with a sedentary lifestyle. The brain-healthy volunteers also had spinal fluid measure consistent with a healthier, amyloid-free brain. So regardless of your genetic predisposition, make an effort to exercise regularly—take a brisk walk, play tennis, swim or do anything that gets your heart to pump oxygen and nutrients to your brain cells.

$Q$: I read that scientists have discovered special immune proteins that attack Alzheimer's plaques in the brain. If those proteins are mass-produce, could that be a new cure?

$A$: These special proteins are called monoclonal anti bodies, and they stimulate an attack on the amyloid plaques associated with Alzheimer's disease. A recent study found that when the proteins were injected into patients with mild to moderate Alzheimer's dementia from two to seven times a month the amount of their brain amyloid decreased by 15 percent compared with patients receiving the placebo injections.

Unfortunately, the patients receiving the proteins did not experience cognitive benefits. The treatment could have been too short to show a clinical effect, or these antibodies may only work for people at risk for dementia, before symptoms of Alzheimer's disease are obvious. To address this theory, prevention trials of these antibodies are currently in progress. Of course, it is also possible that clearing amyloid deposits from the brain is not effective in treating symptoms, and some other approach—fighting tau proteins or curtailing brain inflammation--is more effective.

Q: Lots of people I know have started drinking coconut oil to protect them from Alzheimer's. Do you recommend it?

A: Since Alzheimer's disease has no absolute cure, people are always pursuing new treatments, many based on hope than hope than actual science. In a recent book, a woman described how giving her husband 20 grams of coconut oil twice a day dramatically improved his Alzheimer's symptoms. Based on the idea that an Alzheimer's brain can't get enough glucose into it's cells, providing another source of energy might help those cells get their nutrients and function better. Coconut oil contains fats that the liver converts to ketones, which the brain and other organs can use for energy.

The weakness of the coconut oil theory is that it is based on only one case. It is certainly worth further study, but many nutritionists are concerned about people consuming large amounts coconut oil without any scientific basis since the oil contains saturated fats that can be harmful to heart health. Studies of laboratory animals fed saturated fats shows that they develop high cholesterol levels, increases in brain amyloid and impairment in memory abilities.

Q: I'm becoming addicted to playing *Angry Birds* and other games on my cell phone. My wife says they're ridiculous and childish, but I say they exercise my brain. Who's right?

A: Several studies suggest that playing action video games can improve some cognitive skills. Expert gamers are able to track moving objects at greater speeds and can switch mental tasks more rapidly than non-gamers. However, playing action video games has not been found to improve general cognitive skills involving memory and reasoning. Also, too much fun may not be good for you, especially if you become addicted to the game. You might ask yourself what you are giving up when you spend too much time playing the game. Gaming addiction may draw you away from family, friends, work, and school, so both your personal and professional life might suffer. The key is to balance your *Angry Birds* time with low-teach activities that keep your life in balance, which will likely benefit your brain health, most.

Q: I was taking a lot of over-the-counter herbs and supplements to help my brain power, but my doctor said they don't work and they may be interacting with my blood-thinner medicine. What do you think?

A: Your doctor is partially right. Some supplements do appear to improve brain function when they are tested against placebo. For example, phosphatidylerine, omega-3 fatty acids, vitamin D, $B_6$ and $B_{12}$ and folate have all been found to benefit cognitive abilities compared with placebo in studies lasting several months. However, long-term benefits have not been confirmed. Ginkgo biloba showed positive effects on memory in earlier studies, but the latest large-scale research has not confirmed these benefits. Also ginkgo, as well as vitamin E, can increase the risk for bleeding especially if someone is taking Coumadin or a similar medicine that increases bleeding time.

Just like drug side-effects, the potential adverse effects and interactions from herbal treatments are vast. The stimulating herb ginseng can cause headaches and anxiety. St. John's wort can help some people with depressive symptoms, but it can also interact with antidepressant drugs and some foods to cause side effects ranging from increased blood pressure to nausea and vomiting. You can check out websites (www. personalhealthzone.com/herbsafety html) and other resources that provide details on the side effects and interactions, however it's a good idea to tell your doctor about everything you're taking to ensure that you don't run into problems.

$Q:$ I found a site on the Internet that asks a series of questions and then tells you whether you're getting Alzheimer's disease or not. Can I trust this site?

$A:$ I would not trust any website that claims to be able to make a diagnosis of Alzheimer's disease by answering a series of questions online. A questionnaire can give a doctor information on the degree of memory challenges you are experiencing, but there are many causes of cognitive impairment, ranging from medication side effects to thyroid hormone imbalances. During the course of an evaluation for dementia or Alzheimer's, your doctor may ask a series of questions to determine the extent of cognitive impairment, but several other procedures are necessary. Your doctor needs to ask about your current symptoms and your past medical history. A thorough physical and neurological exam, as well as some laboratory tests, will help determine if a medical illness is contributing to symptoms. An MRI or CT scan is often performed to determine if a stroke or tumor is present, and a PET scan may show a pattern consistent with Alzheimer's disease.

*Q:* I know that a good night's sleep improves my mental focus and energy level, but is there any direct link between sleep and risk for getting Alzheimer's?

*A:* Scientists at Washington University in St. Louis recently discovered that sleep patterns are related to Alzheimer's risk. Amyloid beta, the chemical that forms insoluble brain deposits in Alzheimer's disease, actually declines after about six hours of sleep.

# REFERENCES and WEBSITE RESOURCES

## ALZHEIMER'S ASSOCIATION

919 North Michigan Ave, Suite 1000

Chicago, IL 60611

800-272-3900

www.alz.org

## A SEARCH FOR GOD

ISBN 87604-000-8

Edgar Cayce Readings by

Edgar Cayce Foundation

A.R.E. Press, P.O. 595

Virginia Beach, VA 23451

www.edgarcayce.org

## THE ALZHEIMER'S PREVENTON PROGRAM

Greg Small MD and Gigi Vorgan

ISBN 958-O-7611-7222-2

Workman Publishing Company, Inc.

725 Varick Street

New York, NY 10014-4386

www.workman.com

## HEALTH PROFESSION PRESS

P.O. Box 10624 Baltimore, MD 2 1285-0624

www.healthpropress.com

## BEST FRIENDS

The Best Friends Book of Activities

The Best Friends Approach to Alzheimer's Care

The Best Friends Staff Building

Best Friends (DVD)Video.

www.bestfriendsapproach.com

# Appendix

The author's genealogy consists of Scotch-Irish emigration in the early 19th century to Kentucky and Kansas. His father was a young railroad worker and his mother a waitress in a Fred Harvey railroad restaurant in Winslow, Arizona.

Donald was born on a farm in Kansas about five years after Madge married Henry during the depression. Railroad employment took them to Las Vegas, Nevada to help build Hoover Dam. In 1931, Las Vegas was a small town of 3,000 with gambling and legal prostitution. The family moved to Southern California in 1940 because Henry's job was more secure and his wife got tired of the desert heat. In Southern California, schools were better and Don was happier with a new brother, Bill.

The excitement of World War II led to the family finding air raid wardens, antiaircraft guns and blackouts. One night Angelinos thought they saw Japanese bombers overhead. They later proved to be American planes.

The schools were good for Don and Bill. Progressive education was much better than Las Vegas schools. Don enjoyed singing in high school choir and majored in forestry in junior college.

Don met Penny in Taft, California and they married before he was drafted into the Army for the Korean "Police Action."

Don and Penny went to UCLA with their baby daughter, Melodie, after Don was discharged from the Army.

The university was a series of difficult schedules where our daughter was passed from one of us to the other. We lived in veterans housing on campus and had help from a number of wives of students in our officer barracks apartment. My school time ran from 6:00 to 12:00. I had to meet Penny at 12:30 while she was carrying Melodie onto the athletic field. I would take my daughter back to the apartment and wait until 5:00 PM to greet Penny coming from class. I would then go to my job as janitor in the teaching hospital for the night shift. It's amazing what you can do when you are in your twenties.

School was a great, hard experience. We both made it to graduation in 1957.

I got a vasectomy after David was born when Penny's health began to get complicated from Cushing's disease. I learned all that I could from the teaching hospital's young doctor-students about her condition. One doctor gave the warning that she may not live past 55. I'm glad to report that she lived to be 63 with careful treatment from the best doctors, healers and ministers that I could find, both Catholic and Protestant.

Penny was a speech pathologist and I became a teacher of the handicapped in Orange County. We both worked in state hospitals for the retarded and became "Professionals." Penny developed programs for stutterers and voice disorders.

Penny and I changed our location and positions. Penny started a private practice as a speech pathologist and I became a teacher on educational television in Anaheim.

I learned about an educational media that excluded children from being in my classroom. So I decided to develop scripts, rehearse and present three one-hour social study programs a week at 9 AM on live television. A Ford Foundation grant set up a very effective staff, studio and equipment for my shows that taught mathematics, Spanish, social studies and music to about 5,000; 4th, 5th and 6th graders in Anaheim and later a huge number of children in most Orange County schools.

There were a couple years that the closed-circuit system had no video tape and it was all live. One program about Marco Polo was particularly popular with the students. When I was telling the viewers about Polo's Diary I mistakenly said, "Marco Polo's diarrhea".

I received hundreds of fan letters from 12-year-old students and critical notes and phone calls from teachers who said I had blown up their classrooms.

After that, I taught three more years of *RECORDED* programs and decided that my five year career as a television "star" was over.

I returned to the classroom and was promoted to principal and later an educational manager for the California mental hygiene department over state hospitals.

During summers, I worked at Disneyland as a policeman and I felt a little guilty of taking pay for having so much fun. Disneyland policemen had the job of maintaining peace during operation of the park. That included swimming the river and "rescuing" two teenagers caught having sex at the old fort on an island.

Penny died of Cushing's Syndrome at 63 in 1995 after 30 years of a successful practice and loving life. My daughter, Melodie took me to Venice, Italy to help me get over the loss. I was depressed and felt I wanted to die. Melodie saved my life by taking me out of the gloom of grief.

Eventually I felt like writing a travel book from that experience to help handicapped senior travelers. The book is called, *Venice Easy Sightseeing*. Later, I traveled to Florence and Rome to write a total of three books during the next five years, all for handicapped or senior travelers.

I met my second wife, Ethel, an American traveling in Italy and we became domestic partners back in California at 70 years of age. Ethel was a dog trainer and had a kennel near Bakersfield. She helped me write some of the books and we had a fun marriage until she died of cancer in 2008.

I got mad at God and asked my psychic friend what to do. She said, "I've got good news for you. Your two dead wives have met each other and are watching you. They want to help you." It helped, I found that my next two books had words in them that were not even in my vocabulary. I mopped around between my children; David in St Louis, Missouri with his wife, Charmaine, and my two granddaughters, Erin and Caitlyn. Then I stayed with Melodie, in Napa, California with her husband Cory and my two grandsons, Collin and Quinlan.

Now I reside in a memory care facility, enjoying life and the people who all show me such great care and love.

Made in the USA
San Bernardino, CA
29 October 2015